Intramuscu

By Sharon C Kel

Do you need to give yourself or someone else a "shot" (intramuscular injection)? Has the doctor ordered a medication that can only be given by IM injection? The medication might be vitamin B12, a fertility drug, or maybe some other kind of a hormone. Whatever the medication is, you will need to know how to give it correctly and safely. This book will show you how to do that, and even make you feel comfortable in doing it. I know how apprehensive and intimidated you might feel, because in my years (30) of working as a Registered Nurse, I have experienced those feeling in others and in myself when I first started nursing. I have helped others through their fears. It really is not as difficult as it may seem. OK let's start at the beginning. What do you need to know?

Let's start with supplies!

I suggest that you have a little box or basket even a plastic bag will do, to keep your supplies in. This way, everything that you need will always be together in one place and easy to find. Be sure to keep these supplies out of reach of children. Some medications need to be refrigerated, and in that case the medication will not be kept with the rest of the supplies. Here's what you need:

- Medication vial or ampule (unless kept in the refrigerator)

- Syringes/needles

- Alcohol swabs or bottle of alcohol and cotton balls

- Band-Aids (optional)

- Clean disposable gloves (if you are giving an injection to someone else)

- Puncture proof container for used needle

What should you know about the medication that you are giving?

• What is the name of the medication?

• What is the purpose of the medication?

• How much medication has the doctor ordered?

• How should the medication be stored?

• What are the side effects of the medication?

What should you know about a syringe?

There are three main parts to a syringe: the tip, which connects to the needle, the barrel, or outside part of the syringe, and the plunger, which fits inside the barrel. You must avoid touching or letting anything touch the tip, or inside of the barrel or shaft of the plunger. Only touch the outside of the barrel and the handle of the plunger. Syringes are single use and disposable. Some syringes come with a needle attached and some syringes require you to attach the needle. Syringes are labeled by how much medication they can hold. The syringes used for IM injections have a milliliter scale on them. This scale is marked in tenths (0.1) of milliliters. Make sure the amount of medication you are going to draw up will fit into the syringe you are going to use.

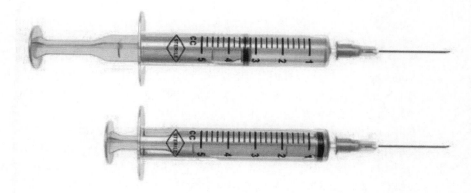

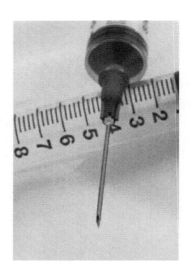

What should you know about a needle?

Needles are labeled by their thickness and length. The package that contains the needle will have 2 numbers on it. The first number will be followed by a G which stands for gauge or thickness of the needle. The higher the number or gauge, the thinner the needle will be. Some medications are thick and therefore need a thicker needle which would be a lower number or gauge.

For an IM injection, the numbers on the needle package will be 21G, 22G, or 23G. The second number on the package is the length of the needle. This will be 1", 1"½", or 2"for an IM injection. The length of the needle is determined by the size of the person getting the injection. The medication is going into a muscle and therefore the needle must be long enough to reach the proper tissue. The doctor or pharmacist will assist you in obtaining the proper size syringe and needle. Also, ask your pharmacist about getting safety needles for your syringes.

After opening the package with the sterile syringe inside, do not touch the tip of the syringe. The tip must remain sterile to attach to the end of the sterile needle. The same is true of the needle. When opening the package, do not touch the uncapped end. If either of these sterile ends touch anything, including your hands, you should dispose of them and get new ones. After attaching the needle to the syringe, lay it down on the inside of the opened syringe package until you are ready to load it with the medication.

Where should I give the injection?

It is important to choose the correct site to inject the medication into for several reasons. First of all, you want to make sure that the medication will be properly absorbed. Also, you want to make sure that you will not cause any injury to yourself or the person you are giving the injection to. An intramuscular injection is given in deep muscle tissue. This is because the muscle can take a larger dose of medication than the loose tissue (subcutaneous) just below the skin can. Also, medications given into muscle tissue are absorbed more quickly. You want a site that is far away from large blood vessels, nerves and bones. In this article, I will show you how to find two different sites that are safe and easy for you to find. They are the ventrogluteal site which is in the hip and the vastus lateralis site which is in the thigh.

The ventrogluteal muscle is located in the hip. This is the site to use if you are giving someone else an injection, not yourself. In order to correctly find and mark the spot for the injection, have the person turn onto their side and bend their knee up toward their chest. This helps to relax the muscle and to see it more easily. However, the person can lie on their back or tummy if they prefer. The first thing you want to do is look at the hip area and make sure there is no bruising or abrasions. Never give an injection in an area that is tender, has a lump, or any kind of tissue injury. In order to correctly find this site, place the palm of your hand over the bony knob at the top, outside thigh (the greater trochanter). Keep your fingers pointing upward toward the person's head. Do this with your right hand if you are going to inject into the left hip. Do this with your left hand if you are going to inject into the right hip. Point your thumb toward the person's groin and your index finger toward the bone at top of buttock (pelvic bone); extend your middle fingerback along the top of the pelvic bone (illiac crest) toward the buttock. The index finger, the middlefinger, and the illiac crest form a V- shaped triangle; the injection site is in the center of the triangle

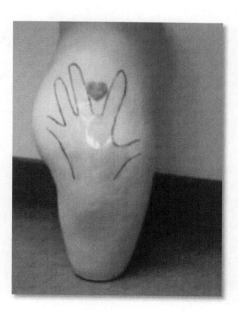

If you are giving yourself an IM injection, use the site that is located in your thigh. This is the vastus lateralis muscle and it is usually thick and well developed in both children and adults. In order to locate the correct spot, divide the front of your thigh into thirds starting at the top of your thigh. You should inject the needle into the middle third slightly toward the outside of the thigh.

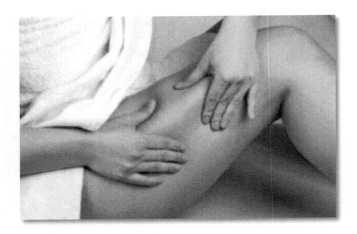

If you choose this area to give an IM injection to someone else, the person can either lie down or sit up for this injection. If the person is obese, this would be the best site to use.

Before you draw the medication up into the syringe, you need to prepare a clean surface to work on and wash your hands.

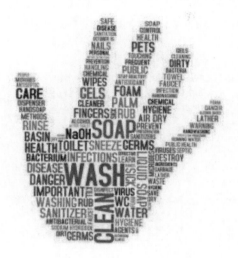

The following steps in handwashing are taken from the CDC website. (Centers for Disease Control)

• Wet your hands with clean, running water (warm or cold) and apply soap.

• Rub your hands together to make lather and scrub them well; be sure to scrub the backs of your hands, between your fingers, and under your nails

• Continue rubbing your hands for at least 20 seconds. (hum the "Happy Birthday" song from beginning to end twice).

• Rinse your hands well under running water.

• Dry your hands using a clean towel or air dry them.

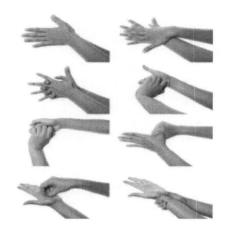

Note: washing hands with soap and water is the best way to reduce the number of germs on them. If soap and water are not available, use an alcohol-based hand sanitizer that contains at least 60% alcohol. Alcohol-based hand sanitizers can quickly reduce the number of germs on hands in some situations, but sanitizers do **not** eliminate all types of germs.

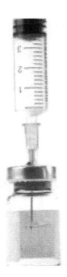

How to draw up medication from a vial and an ampule!

• Check the name on the vial of medication to make sure it is for the person you are going to give the injection too.

• Check the expiration date on the vial to make sure the medication hasn't expired.

• Look to see how many mls are in the vial.   Do you have enough medication?

• If the vial has not been opened, remove the metal cap.

 • Wipe the rubber top in a circular motion with an alcohol pad and let it dry.

• While the vial top is drying, pick up the syringe touching only the outside of the barrel and the handle of the plunger. • Remove the cap from the needle and draw up air into the syringe equal to the amount of medication that you will withdraw from the medication vial.

• Very carefully insert the needle into the center of the rubber cap of the vial. Be careful not to let the needle touch anything except the rubber cap.

• Inject the air into the vial (this makes it easier to withdraw the medication) keeping the tip (bevel) of the needle above the surface of the medication so bubbles are not created.

• Withdraw the correct amount of medication by inverting the vial, keeping the tip of the syringe below the fluid level, and holding the vial and syringe at eye level.

 • Eject any air that might be at the top of the syringe and withdraw the needle from the vial.

• Carefully replace the cap over the needle. Do not let the needle touch anything.

• Eject any air bubbles from the syringe by gently tapping on the barrel of the syringe with your finger or a pen while holding the syringe with the needle end pointing up.

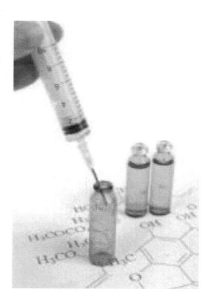

If the medication comes in an ampule, you will need a filter needle to draw up the medication. This is because tiny bit of glass could get into the medication while snapping off the top. Before snapping off the prescored neck of the ampule, tap the top of the ampule with your finger until all of the fluid is out of the neck. Place an unopened alcohol swab around the neck of the ampule and snap the top off away from your hands. Put the filter needle on your syringe and draw up the medication out of the ampule.   Hold the ampule upside down or set it on a flat surface. Insert the filter needle down into the center of the ampule into the fluid without touching the rim of the ampule. Draw the medication up into the syringe by pulling back on the plunger keeping the tip of the needle under the surface of the liquid. If you see air bubbles, take the needle out of the ampule and hold the syringe with the needle pointing up. Tap the side of the syringe to expel the air bubbles. Cover the filter needle with its cap and then remove it from the syringe. Replace the filter needle with a non filter needle for the injection.

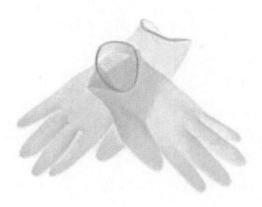

Let's give the injection!

• If you are giving an injection to someone else, put on a pair of clean, disposable gloves.

• Make sure the sharps container is nearby so that you can dispose of the used needle immediately after the injection.

• Clean the site with an alcohol swab by starting in the center and rotating outward in a circular motion for about 2 inches.

• Let the site dry. Do not blow on it or fan it dry. This just puts germs back on the site.

• Apply pain medication cream (optional)

• Remove the needle cover by pulling it straight off. If you twist it, it may come loose from the syringe and fall off.

• Hold the syringe between your thumb and forefinger of your dominant hand. Hold syringe like a dart – palm down.

• Spread the skin to one side with the side of your non - dominate hand and hold your hand there until the medication is injected. This insures that the medication gets into the tissue.

• With dominate hand inject needle quickly like a dart (90 degree angle)

• Before injecting the medication and while continuing to hold the skin to the side with your non – dominate hand, stabilize the barrel with that same hand so that you can draw back slightly on the plunger with your dominate hand to see if any blood comes back into the syringe. If no blood, then inject the medication slowly into the muscle while still holding the skin to the side. Pull the needle out steadily before releasing the skin.

• Another option is to grasp the body of the muscle between your thumb and forefinger with your non – dominate hand and then with your dominant hand, inject the needle quickly at a 90 degree angle into the muscle (like a dart). Again, stabilize the barrel with the same hand that you are holding the muscle with and with your other hand, pull back slightly on the plunger to see if any blood comes back into the syringe. If you do not see any blood, inject the medication slowly into the muscle. Before releasing the skin, pull the needle out steadily.

• Apply gentle pressure over the site with a gauze or alcohol swab. Do not massage the site. Apply a band aid if needed.

•Discard the uncapped needle into sharps container

• Remove gloves and dispose of them in a waste container.

• Wash your hands.

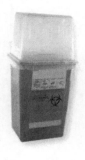

If you do not have a sharps container like one shown here, you can use a hard, plastic bottle that you cannot see through. A detergent bottle would work fine.

Giving an injection takes some practice, so before you give that first one, practice all the steps on someone without a needle on the syringe.

Also, you might wonder why you are checking for blood in the syringe before you inject the medication. This is because, if blood does come back up into the syringe and you go ahead and give the injection, you would be injecting the medication into a blood vessel instead of the muscle and this could be dangerous.

If you see blood in the plunger of the syringe what should you do? You should **stop**. Do not inject the medication but instead pull out the needle and dispose of the syringe, medication and all, into the sharps container and start all over with new supplies. This does not happen very often. It has happened to me once in all my years of practice

Some additional tips to consider when giving an intramuscular injection!

• Injections do hurt but there are some things you can do to deal with this. You can use ice to numb the area before cleaning with alcohol.
• Rotate the sites you give the injection into. Switch from one hip to the other or one thigh to the other. Also, never inject medication into the same exact spot repeatedly because this can cause tissue damage.
• There is a pain relieving cream that the doctor can order to apply to the site a few minutes before the injection is going to be given.
• Try to relax the muscle. Tension in the muscle makes the injection more painful.
• If you are injecting an oil-based medication, massage the site after the injection. This can help the medication to absorb faster.
• After drawing up the medication, change the needle. The needle you have drawn the medication up with has been dulled going through the rubber stopper of the vial.

When to Call the Doctor

- Redness at the injection site that does not go away.
- Warmth at the injection site that does not go away.
- Swelling or hardness under the skin that does not go away.
- Drainage at the site especially if it has color to it or has an odor.
  - Fever greater than 101 that cannot be related to something else.
- Severe pain that does not go away (some pain is expected)

Resource List

www.caregiver.com

www.caregiversupportnetwork.org

www.caringinfo.org/caringforsomeone

www.helpguide.org/elder/caring_for_caregivers.htm

About the author:

Sharon Kelly is a Registered Nurse who is currently working in the Nursing Department of a Community College. She has done hospital nursing, home health & hospice nursing, and nursing education. Please visit her websites:

www.skillsfornurses.com

www.thehomecarer.com

.

Printed in Great Britain
by Amazon.co.uk, Ltd.,
Marston Gate.